Cover Design:
Photograph of a unique lacquer technique
developed by Only Definitive Designs.

Interior Illustration:
Digital rendering of an original painting entitled:
"Bambooxia" 1978
Luma dyes with French quill brush on waxed massa rice paper.
Artist-Luanne Ward

ISBN-13: 978-0998883946 (Artistic Engine, LLC)

ISBN-10: 0998883948

www.ArtisticEngine.com

(631) UNLEASH (631) 865-3274

www.OnlyDefDesigns.com

Give Voice To Your Spirit

Name

Written & Illustrated
by
Luanne Ward

"Give Voice To Your Spirit" is a book with simple questions that guide you, as you write about your life.

An "inheritance" for your family.
An inheritance of your *TRUE* wealth.
The wealth of spirit, heart and strength that lives in your story.

Create a lasting document.
Including all kinds of information,
thoughts and stories.
A document of your life, spirit and personality.

Build a foundation
for future generations to build on.

Give your children a connection to the past.
Without documents, pictures and stories,
in just two generations, we can forget.

One of the most powerful things we can do,
to enrich the lives of our family for generations to come,
is to plant a family "TREE".

Cultivate it until it has lots of leaves, strong branches
and clearly defined roots.

A legacy is built over time.

The time is now!

Start with this. Start today.

Tomorrow is promised to no one.

Infuse these pages with love, honesty, humor and hope.
Write as much or as little as you choose.
Include the good and the not-so-good. Have fun with it.

On a commuter train, during your lunch hour, while on vacation or
during the commercial of your favorite TV show.
Take every and any opportunity to add information.

Feel free to change or modify the writing suggestions
or add topics of your own.

Once you have added all your information,
memories, & experiences
we provide an extra special service.

For an additional fee, you can return the completed book to us
and we will publish duplicate copies of your finished book.

This unique service allows you to give each of your children & family members their own professionally printed and bound copy of your finished book.
You can even add pictures during the duplication process.

There are two books in this series.
The companion book is entitled
"A Voice Remembered"
a book that guides several family members & friends as they write about ***a loved-one's life***.
www.AVoiceRemembered.com

Families come in all shapes and sizes.
Sometimes biology is included.
Other times, the human spirit alone, holds the connection.

Our hope is to inspire you to establish a tradition,
of documenting ***your family history***.

Words, pictures, videos, every way you can!

Shining light on the past, gives light to the future.
What we do to strengthen our families today,
will strengthen the human family tomorrow.

Mother to daughter, father to son, cousin to cousin
or friend to friend. However you choose to share it,
share it with love & good cheer.

The connection, the word -FAMILY- implies, is an
((((((((((((((energy))))))))))))))).
It is up to each of us to do what we can,
to generate and preserve it.

TABLE OF CONTENTS

TABLE OF CONTENTS (continued)

TABLE OF CONTENTS (continued)

TABLE OF CONTENTS (continued)

TABLE OF CONTENTS (continued)

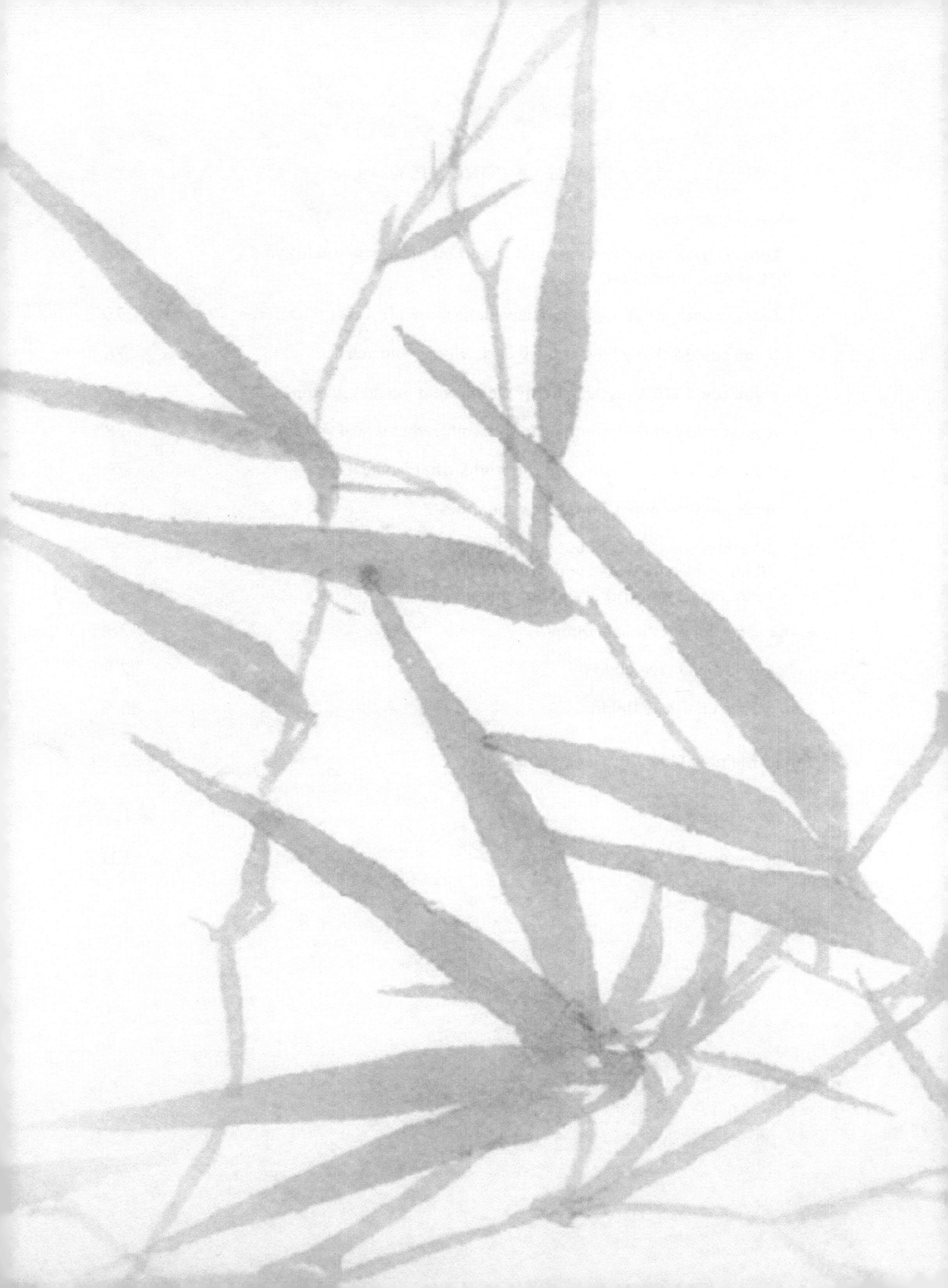

Chapter 1

Background

What is your full, given name?

Date of birth?

Time of day you were born?

Day of the week you were born?

Where were you born?

What do you know about the day you were born, days/weeks leading up to your birth.

Where is your family originally from?

Where did you live growing up?

Who did you live with?

What are some physical traits in your family?

Personality traits?

What did your parents do for a living?

Jobs they had through the years?

What is something you want people to know about your family?

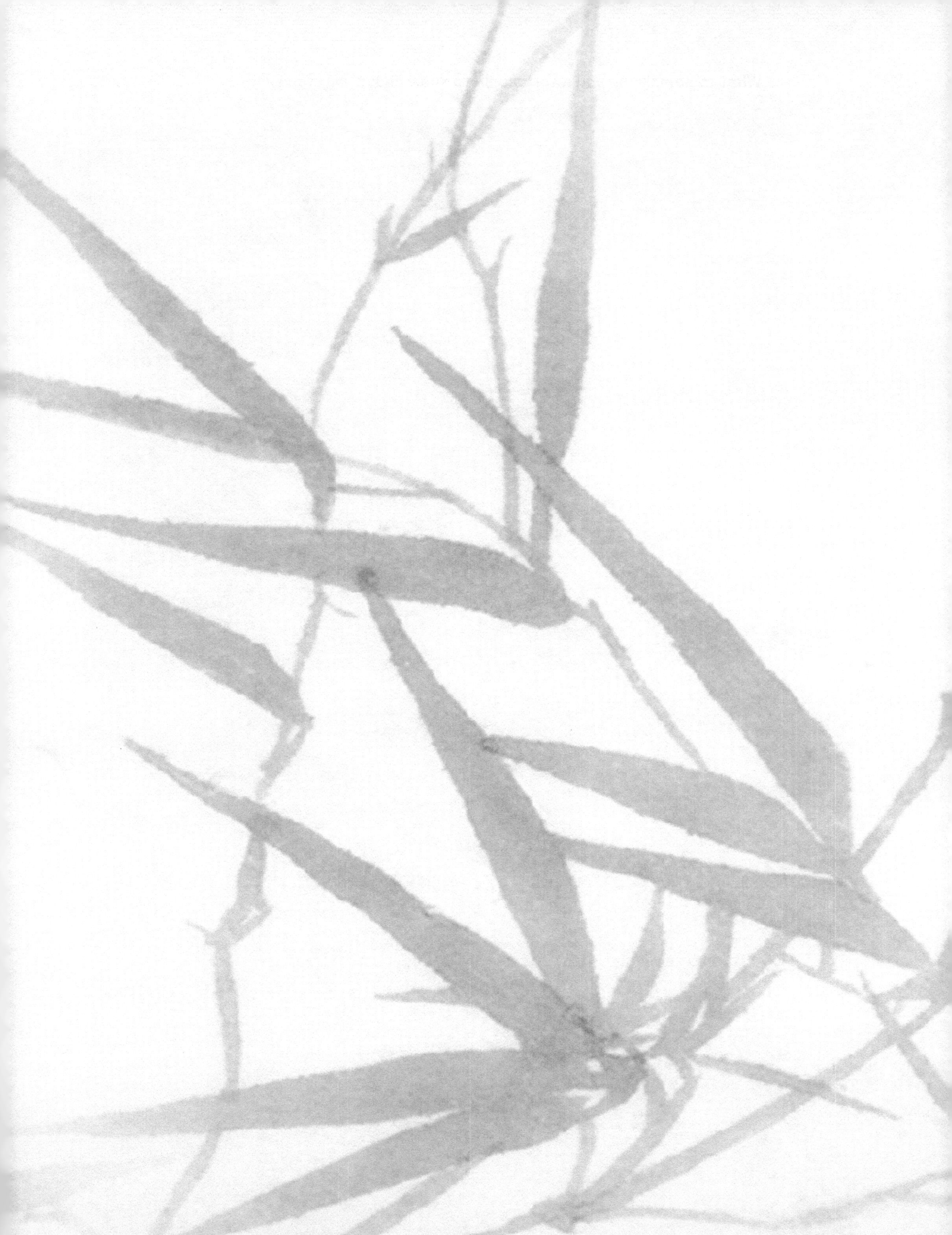

Chapter 2

Family & Friends

Mother's Name:

Tell me about your mother.

Father's Name:

Tell me about your father.

Tell me about your brothers and sisters.

Tell me about your grandparents on your mother's side of your family.

Tell me about your grandparents on your father's side of your family.

Tell me about your children.

Tell me about your grandchildren.

Tell me about other members of your family. Nieces, Nephews, Aunts, Uncles, Cousins.

Tell me about your close family friends.

Chapter 3

Growing Up

What were you like as a child?

Did you have a nickname? Who gave it to you, and why?

Who were your best friends growing up?

What did you want to be growing up?

Who did you look up to when you were young?

Tell me about the house(s) or apartment(s) you lived in through the years.

Tell me about the neighborhood(s) you've lived in.

Tell me about memorable people in your community.

What was a typical day like as a child?

What did you fight about with your brother(s), sister(s) or friend(s)?

Tell me about a time, you got into trouble as a child.

Tell me about a time, you got into trouble as a teenager.

What were you afraid of, growing up?

What did you worry about growing up?

How did you overcome some of your childhood fears and worries?

What did your family do in the evening or on weekends for entertainment?

What did you like to do when you had time to yourself when you were young?

On an average day, (as a child/as a teenager) what did you do after school?

What were the popular trends or new inventions when you were young?

Tell me about pets you've had through the years.

If you drive, how old were you when you first got your license?

How do you feel about driving?

What kinds of cars have you driven through the years?

Tell me about a memorable driving or riding experience.

Tell me something about boyfriends/girlfriends you had through the years.

Tell me about the first time you went on a date. Memorable dates.

Chapter 4

Favorites

What were your favorite things to do when you were a child?

What were your favorite things to do as a teenager?

What were your favorite color(s) as a young person?

What are your favorite color(s) now?

To wear?

For a vehicle?

For a room?

What hair styles have you worn through the years?

How would you describe your "style"?

Tell me which you prefer and Why?

Silver or gold?

Slippers or barefoot?

Warm weather or cold weather?

Elvis or The Beetles?

Watch TV or read?

Go to a concert or go to a sporting event?

Night life or camping?

Playing sports or playing video games?

Cats or dogs?

Birds or fish?

Tell me your favorites:

Music:

Movies:

Television Shows:

Books:

Magazines:

Websites:

Foods:

Beverages:

Tell me some things you really don't like and why?

What are your Hobbies? Now and as a child.

Chapter 5

Education/Career/Jobs

What schools did you attend?

How did you feel about school?

What was your favorite subject or class?

Who was your favorite teacher(s)?

What was your first job? How old were you?

Tell me about jobs you had through the years.

Which of your accomplishments are you most proud of?

What challenge taught you the most?

Chapter 6

Influences & Beliefs

What are your spiritual beliefs?

How have your beliefs developed through the years?

What basic values do you live by?

Through the years, how has life surprised you?

Who has had the greatest influence on who you are today or how you live your life?

What event had the greatest influence on who you are today or how you live your life?

What holidays did you celebrate growing up? How did you celebrate them?

Tell me about your most memorable holiday moment.

What advice would you like to pass along?

What advice do you wish you had taken?

What advice do you wish you had ignored?

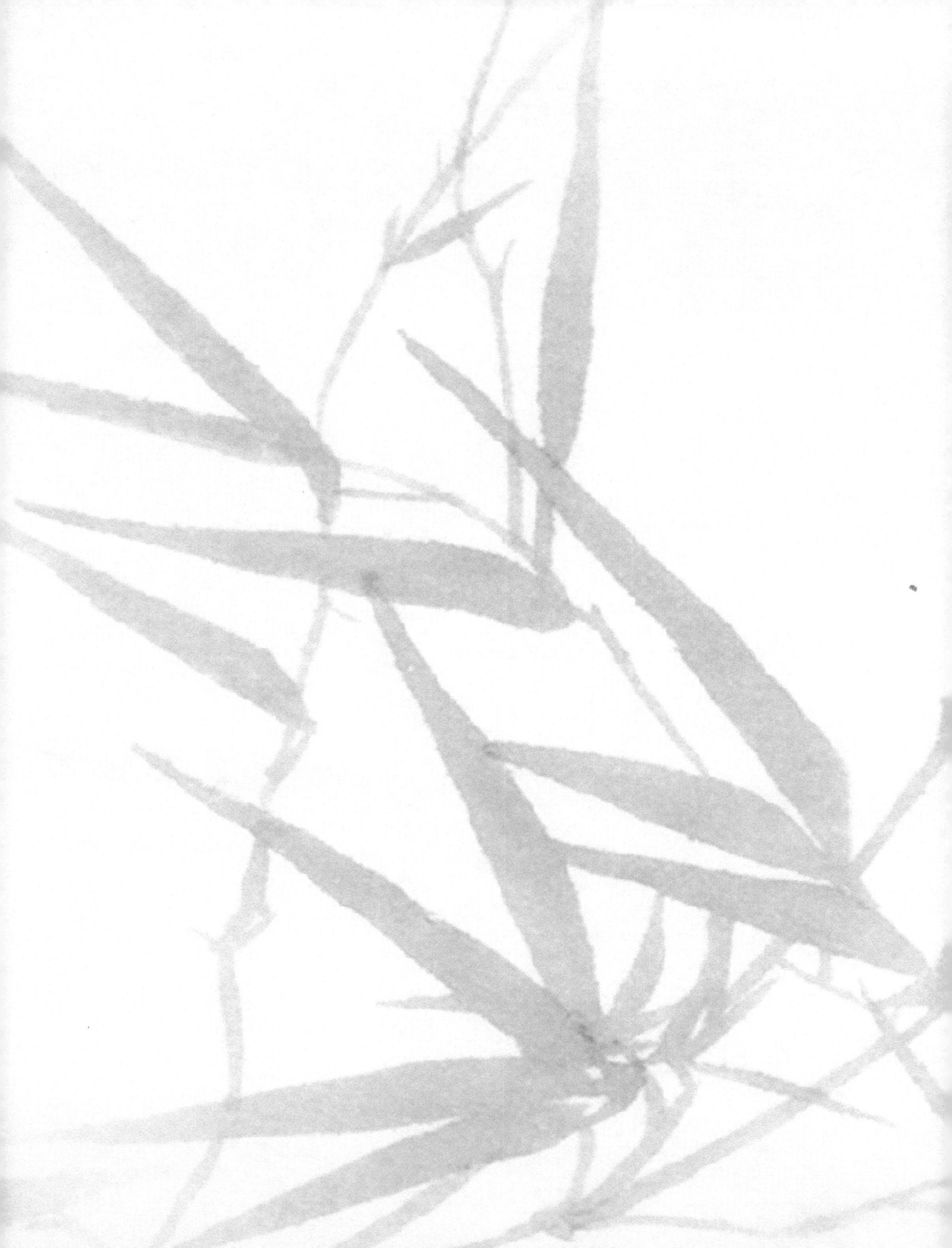

Chapter 7

Now

How did you meet your significant other?

What do you like to do when you have time for yourself now?

What was a hard lesson you had to learn?

What scares or worries you today?

What brings you the greatest joy in your life?

What are some family traditions you hope will continue?

Tell me about a time, you think of as, one of the best days of your life?

Tell me about a time, you think of as, one of the worst days of your life?

What inventions we have today, could you never have imagined, growing up?

Which new invention(s) changed your life the most?

Looking back, what was the most important life lesson you learned?

How does it help you?

Looking back, what might you have done MORE of?

LESS of?

DIFFERENTLY?

If you could DO anything in the world, what would you do?

If you could STOP anything in the world, what would you stop?

If you could CHANGE anything in the world, what would you change?

If you could HAVE anything in the world, what would it be?

What are your hopes for future generations?

Did you enjoy writing about your life?

When and where would you write?

What impact did writing and remembering have on you?

continued from page:___________

continued from page:

continued from page:___________

continued from page:

continued from page:___________

continued from page:__________

continued from page:___________

continued from page:

continued from page:___________

continued from page:

INSTRUCTIONS:
Start with the name of the person you are documenting.

Fill in the name of their Mother and Father .

List each brother/sister's name - the names of their children and the names of their grandchildren.
Add facts about marriage, birthdays, etc..

Families are complicated!
Feel free to add to or change the format as necessary.

Only Definitive Designs New York
Unleashing Creativity

BROTHER/SISTER'S GRANDCHILDREN

BROTHER/SISTER'S GRANDCHILDREN

GRANDCHILDREN

BROTHER/SISTER'S CHILDREN

BROTHER/SISTER'S CHILDREN

CHILDREN

BROTHER/SISTER

BROTHER/SISTER

NAME

MOTHER

FATHER

INSTRUCTIONS:
Start with the name of the person you are documenting.

Fill in the name of their Mother and Father .

List each brother/sister's name - the names of their children and the names of their grandchildren.
Add facts about marriage, birthdays, etc..

Families are complicated!
Feel free to add to or change the
format as necessary.

Only Definitive Designs New York
Unleashing Creativity

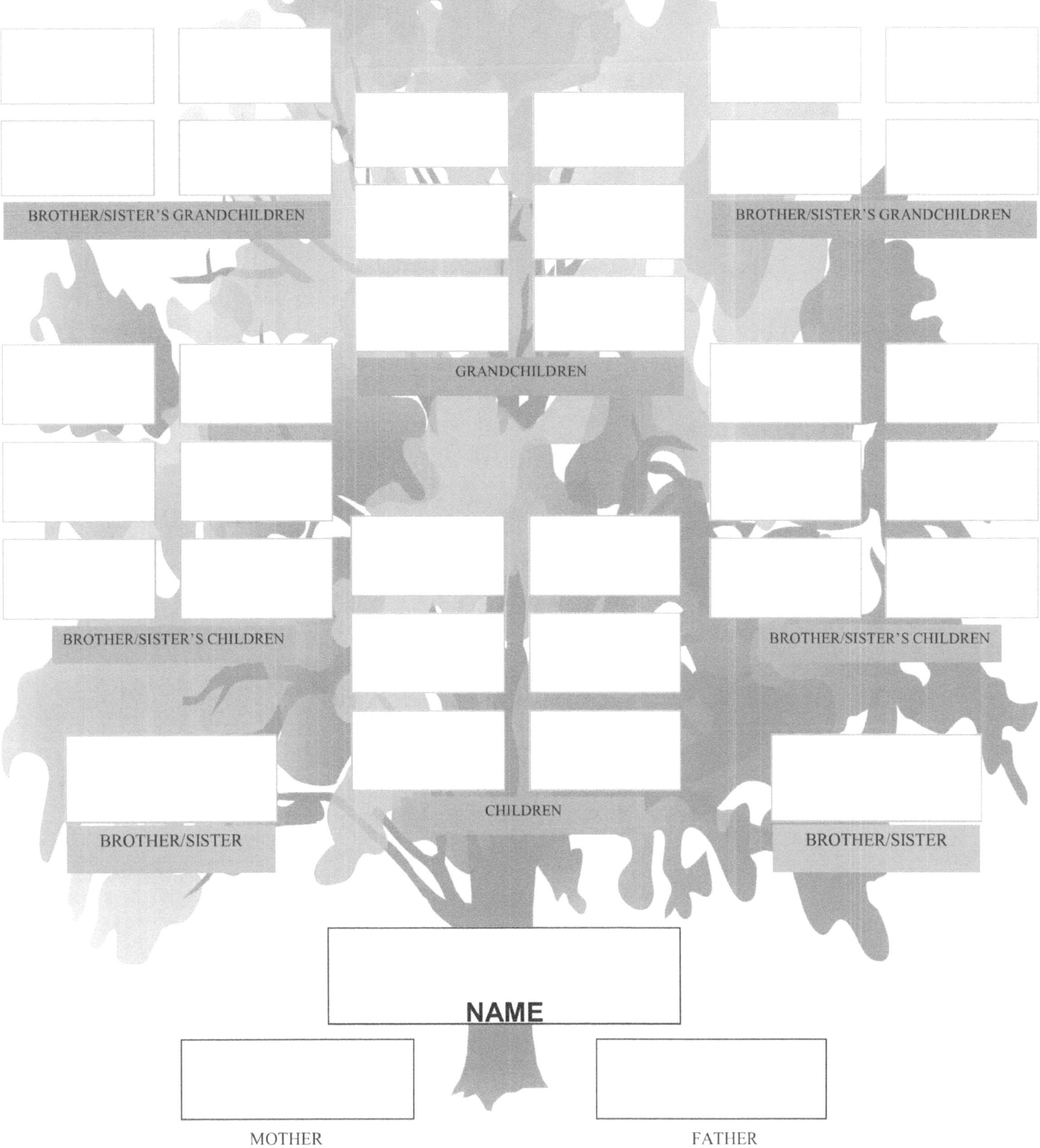

INSTRUCTIONS:
Start with the name of the person you are documenting.

Fill in the name of their Mother and Father .

List each brother/sister's name - the names of their children and the names of their grandchildren.
Add facts about marriage, birthdays, etc..

Families are complicated!
Feel free to add to or change the format as necessary.

Only Definitive Designs New York
Unleashing Creativity

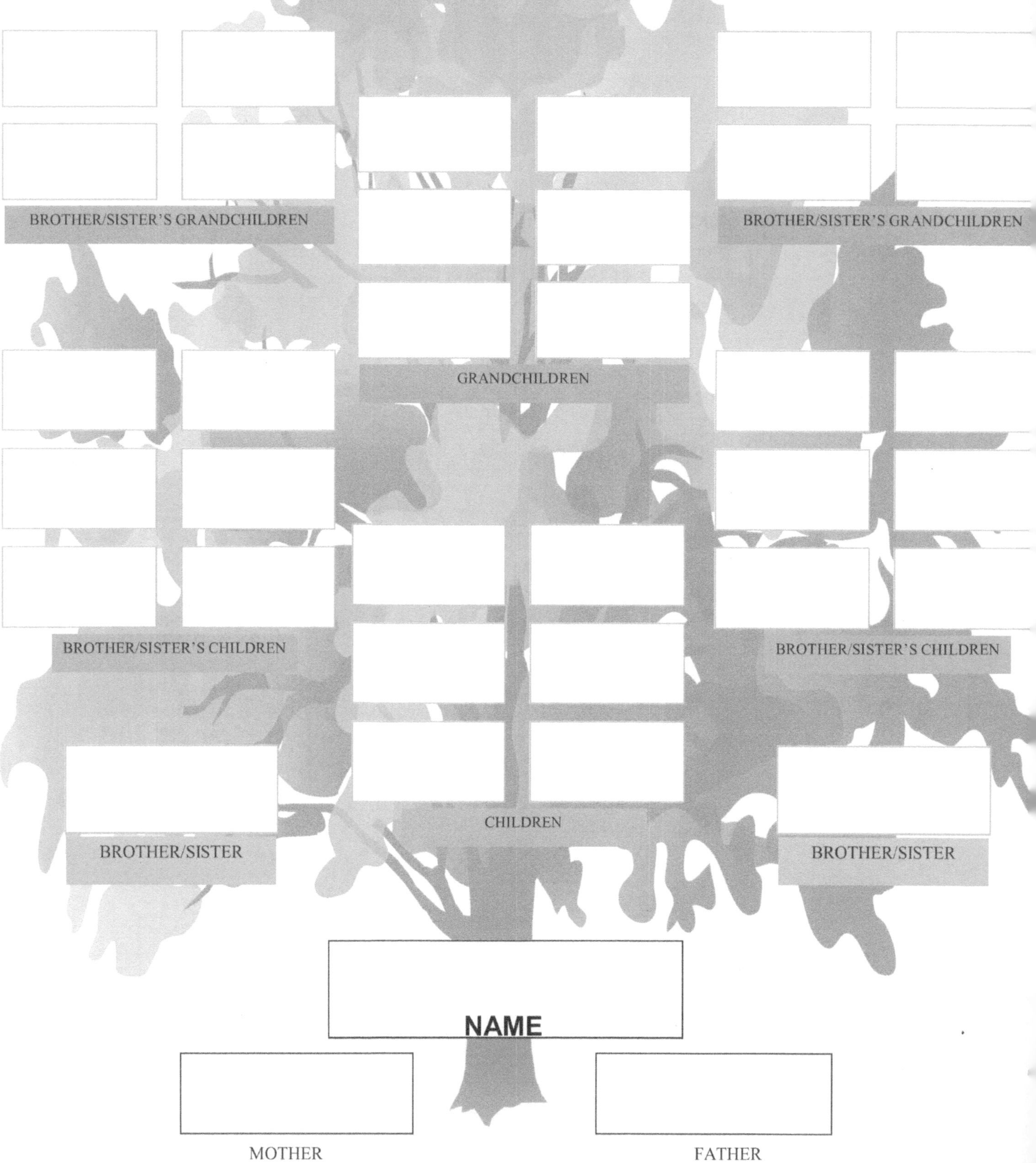

INSTRUCTIONS:
This Family Tree Chart is designed to detail family from a particular union or marriage.

Add as much as you know about each family member. Birth dates, accomplishments, etc.

Families are complicated!
Feel free to add to or change the format as need.

ONLY Definitive Designs New York
Unleashing Creativity

Grandchild / Birth Date

Grandchild / Birth Date

Grandchild / Birth Date

Grandchild / Birth Date

Grandchild / Birth Date

Grandchild / Birth Date

Child / Birth Date

Child / Birth Date

Child / Birth Date

From the union/marriage of:

Partner/Spouse/Mate NAME - Birth Date

Partner/Spouse/Mate NAME - Birth Date

Marriage information - when, where and dates. Where they lived together. Where they lived growing up. Their parents names. Occupations. etc.

INSTRUCTIONS:
This Family Tree Chart is designed to detail family from a particular union or marriage.

Add as much as you know about each family member. Birth dates, accomplishments, etc.

Families are complicated!
Feel free to add to or change the format as need.

Only Definitive Designs New York
Unleashing Creativity

Grandchild / Birth Date

Grandchild / Birth Date

Grandchild / Birth Date

Grandchild / Birth Date

Grandchild / Birth Date

Grandchild / Birth Date

Child / Birth Date

Child / Birth Date

Child / Birth Date

From the union/marriage of:

Partner/Spouse/Mate NAME - Birth Date

Partner/Spouse/Mate NAME - Birth Date

Marriage information - when, where and dates. Where they lived together. Where they lived growing up. Their parents names. Occupations. etc.

INSTRUCTIONS:
This Family Tree Chart is designed to detail family from a particular union or marriage.

Add as much as you know about each family member. Birth dates, accomplishments, etc.

Families are complicated! Feel free to add to or change the format as need.

ONLY Definitive Designs New York
Unleashing Creativity

Grandchild / Birth Date

Grandchild / Birth Date

Grandchild / Birth Date

Grandchild / Birth Date

Grandchild / Birth Date

Grandchild / Birth Date

Child / Birth Date

Child / Birth Date

Child / Birth Date

From the union/marriage of:

Partner/Spouse/Mate NAME - Birth Date

Partner/Spouse/Mate NAME - Birth Date

Marriage information - when, where and dates. Where they lived together. Where they lived growing up. Their parents names. Occupations. etc.

INSTRUCTIONS:
This Family Tree Chart is designed to detail family living in a particular geographical area.

Add as much as you know about each family member.

Family members living in:

Location

Name / Birth Date

Address
Mother's Name
Father's Name
Spouse
Children's Names

Occupation
Other Information

Name / Birth Date

Address
Mother's Name
Father's Name
Spouse
Children's Names

Occupation
Other Information

Name / Birth Date

Address
Mother's Name
Father's Name
Spouse
Children's Names

Occupation
Other Information

Name / Birth Date

Address
Mother's Name
Father's Name
Spouse
Children's Names

Occupation
Other Information

INSTRUCTIONS:
This Family Tree Chart is designed to detail family living in a particular geographical area.

Add as much as you know about each family member.

Family members living in:

Location

Only Definitive Designs New York
Unleashing Creativity

Name / Birth Date

Address
Mother's Name
Father's Name
Spouse
Children's Names

Occupation
Other Information

Name / Birth Date

Address
Mother's Name
Father's Name
Spouse
Children's Names

Occupation
Other Information

Name / Birth Date

Address
Mother's Name
Father's Name
Spouse
Children's Names

Occupation
Other Information

Name / Birth Date

Address
Mother's Name
Father's Name
Spouse
Children's Names

Occupation
Other Information

The Author's Notes

The inspiration and catalyst for this book series, Book One~"Give Voice To Your Spirit" and Book Two~"Voices Remembered", was the traumatic lose of five family members in a matter of months. My only Aunt, my son's Father (who was the love of my life). The day we buried him, my Grandmother passed. A few weeks latter my Father transcended. Then my cousin, at only 59 years old.

Losing five family members within such a short period of time, left me no time to grieve or recover. I had work to do. As the family Artist, I lovingly designed each funeral program. Sorting through hundreds of pictures, formatting and re-formatting the obituaries and processionals. Reading and re-reading poems, scriptures and passages that would convey an authentic expression of their lives.

I wanted to do my BEST for each of them. I wanted each person, who came to pay their respects, to in-a-glance, have a feeling of the whole life of my loved-one. I included pictures of them throughout their lives and personalized each with images that conveyed the best of who they were in life.

I wanted each program to personify beauty and grace. I wanted all who received the programs to be able to see, they had been produced with love. Each program was printed by hand on high-end specialty papers and had multiple pages. Each was laced by hand with satin ribbon, silver and gold cord.

Although the experience was draining, it intensified my understanding of just how fragile life is. I came away wanting to create something more substantial than a program that would be placed in a drawer or thrown away. I was compelled to find a way for everyone to create a "fitting" tribute to their family members. A tribute that would stand the test of time and be available to future generations. That is the inspiration that created this book series.

Book One ~"Give Voice To Your Spirit" came first. I wanted to create an easy way for everyone to write down a few remarks about their life.

Then came, Book Two ~"A Voice Remembered". Designed to allow several family members and friends to honor and document the life, spirit and energy of a loved-one. To capture their personality and preserve it. An invaluable reference, for future generations. A connection to their heritage.

I began to consider, what it is, to leave an inheritance for my family. Inheritance is defined in the dictionary as - a valued possession which is passed down through generations; a permanent or valuable possession or blessing, received by an heir from an ancestor; especially one received as a gift; a benefaction.

The greatest gift I have received from my ancestors is, the hope and spirit that lives in their stories. Writing these stories down, creates a permanent and valuable possession. An inheritance of my family's TRUE wealth, our spirit.

This is my effort, to help make it easier for everyone to begin establishing an inheritance for their families. To help document the connections that bind us together as a family, Past, Present & Future.

I wish Peace & Blessings to you and yours, Always!
Luanne Ward.

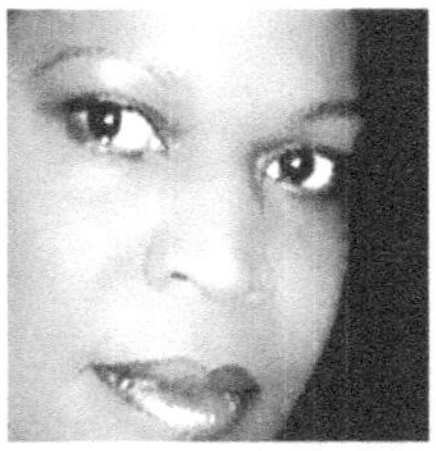

I am an Artist.
I was born
this way.
It's not just
what I do,
it's what I am.

About the Author

Luanne Ward is an Artist. Born in Queens, NY. One of her first memories is from nursery school. She remembers her teacher Mrs. Watson, proclaiming, "Give the decorations to Luanne, she's the creative one." Growing up, her creativity was acknowledged by many people in her life. Art and dance lessons as a child, fine art major in high school, and while doing course work at Parsons: School of Design and The New School For Social Research, she spent her free time as stage manager, costume and scenic designer to New York's dance and theatrical performance groups.

Ms. Ward is the founder and lead artist of Only Definitive Designs, a design strategy company, offering creative presentation solutions to a range of industries. One tag line for her company reads: *Presentation is Everything.* Like she always says, "You can have the best product in the world, but if it is not presented well, no one will ever know about it." The company specializes in creative products including electronic press kits, promotional packages, flash movies, websites, CD & DVD covers, posters, logos, brochures, flyers and business cards.

Her film industry credits include: Set Designer on the award winning film "Silent Cries of A Child". A film adaptation of a poem about child abuse. Written by Lisa V. Stokes. Directed by Iris Goodwin. Also winning awards is "A Deeper Love". A faith-based film about the strength of love. Written and Directed by Darrell Smith. Lawrence Layne Productions came to her to create a cover design and poster that would take this film to the next level. She did just that. Set Designer, as well as Cover Designer on "Choices". A film created for the Administration For Children's Services, Directed by Iris Goodwin. This powerful film is seen by young people as an important part of many city and state programs.

Luanne Ward authored her first book, "Through The Eyes Of My Sister", was inspired by the magical experience she had in response to her sister's missionary journey to South Africa. Artistically designed and illustrated with full color artwork and photos. A portion of the proceeds from this literary work go to benefit the people of South Africa.

In response to the need for arts in her community, Ms. Ward established a mobile arts center providing quality arts education wherever the need exists. "Unleashing Creativity" is the tag line for this venture. Dynamic workshop series and day events, transform an ordinary space into an art studio. Community organizations, hospitals, day habilitation centers, schools, churches, you name it*!* Participants create personalized, fine handcrafts & artwork. Specialized techniques and tools allow people, of all ages and abilities, to create high-end art pieces with professional finishes. These workshops create a natural path to creative fund raising events and campaigns.

Ms. Ward is also the Director of a Supplemental Educational Service program supporting Public Schools and works as an Art Therapist helping to develop the artistic expression of young adults with Autism.

www.OnlyDDny.com ▪ www.CLiPsDVD.com ▪ www.OnlyDefDesigns.com
www.AVoiceRemembered.com ▪ www.GiveVoice2YourSpirit.com

Made in United States
Cleveland, OH
05 November 2026

47663577R00065